HOSPITAL ARTS
A Sound Approach

Rosalie Rebollo Pratt, Ed.D., BCIAC

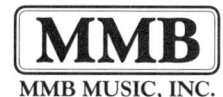

MMB MUSIC, INC.

HOSPITAL ARTS
A Sound Approach

Rosalie Rebollo Pratt, Ed.D., BCIAC

© Copyright 1997 MMB Music, Inc. All rights reserved. International protection secured under Berne, UCC, Buenos Aires and bilateral copyright treaties. No part of this publication may be reproduced, stored in a retrieval system, or transmitted—in any form or by any means now known or later developed—without prior written permission except in the case of brief quotations embodied in critical articles and reviews.

Cover photo: Alan Groesbeck, Media Specialist, Utah Valley Regional Medical Center
On cover: Ronald A. Stoddard, M.D., Codirector, Newborn Intensive Care, Unit, Utah Valley Regional Medical Center, Provo, Utah; an infant in the Premature Intensive Care Unit; and Jacquelyn M. Coleman, M.A., Codirector, Hospital Arts Program, Provo, Utah.
Typography: Gary K. Lee
Printer: Patterson Printing, Benton Harbor, MI
1st printing: October 1997
Printed in USA
ISBN: 0-918812-97-6

For further information and catalogs contact:

MMB Music, Inc.
Contemporary Arts Building
3526 Washington Avenue
Saint Louis, MO 63103-1019 USA

Phone: 314 531-9635, 800 543-3771 (USA/Canada)
Fax: 314 531-8384
E-mail: mmbmusic@mmbmusic.com
Web site: http://www.mmbmusic.com

for George

CONTENTS

Foreword   vi

Introduction   vii

Chapter 1
    The Creative Arts in Healthcare: An Idea Whose Time Has Come   1

Chapter 2
    How to Incorporate the Creative Arts in a Hospital Environment   6

Chapter 3
    The Creative Arts in a Private Practice   13

Chapter 4
    Music and the Other Creative Arts for the Elderly   17

Chapter 5
    People in Crisis or Difficult Circumstances   21

Chapter 6
    Fund Raising and Research   26

Chapter 7
    Basic Resources, Promotion, and Assessment   32

Chapter 8
    Four Models of Hospital Arts Programs   38

FOREWORD

Art Access/Very Special Arts Utah is an affiliate of Very Special Arts, which was founded in 1974 by Jean Kennedy Smith as a program of the John F. Kennedy Center for the Performing Arts in Washington, D.C. Our nonprofit organization is part of a vital network of Very Special Arts organizations that span 50 states and more than 86 countries around the world.

Serving over 17,000 individuals statewide each year, Art Access/Very Special Arts Utah provides quality arts programming and experiences for children and adults with disabilities, and other underserved individuals. We seek to promote the abilities of all persons through the positive and often healing power of the arts.

Our relationship with Dr. Rosalie Rebollo Pratt has been long and productive, and we are proud to sponsor the Hospital Arts Program at Brigham Young University under her able leadership. Since it is well documented that the human spirit responds positively to the creative arts, it makes perfect sense that the arts be afforded a respected place in hospital and institutional settings.

We heartily invite you to read *Hospital Arts: A Sound Approach*. Both inspiring and practical, this lovingly written book provides the tools and know-how of those who have successfully toiled in the field of arts and healthcare. We hope that you will embrace the possibilities presented and adapt them to your own needs and healthcare situation. You can be assured of the rewards inherent in implementing the programs described in the text or in similar programs of your own design. Both you as healthcare professionals and/or volunteers, and those individuals whom you care for in a hospital or institutional setting, will reap the very real benefits of integrating the arts into the healing process.

                              Ruth Lubbers
                              Executive Director
                              Art Access/Very Special Arts Utah

INTRODUCTION

This manual is written for anyone interested in a cost-effective program for integrating the creative arts in the healthcare environment, including but not limited to performing artists, creative arts therapists, hospital and medical office staff, physicians, nurses, administrators, community volunteers, and social workers. The intent is to offer a model to artists and laypersons alike for incorporating the creative arts in healthcare facilities and physicians' offices.

Creative arts therapists provide a very specific and highly trained service to patients, individually and in groups. This manual suggests a program involving musicians, artists, and others not necessarily trained in any formal therapy program. The proposed plan augments (but does not replace) professionally trained therapists' services by involving creative arts majors and community volunteers in providing live instrumental and vocal music, storytelling, dance, drama, and the other creative arts to patients in small and large groups. The plan in no way involves any formal therapeutic approach, which is of course the domain of professionals trained in these techniques. What it does provide is the gift of the arts as a way of humanizing the hospital and office environments and bringing people together in creative arts activities. The ideas are simple enough to be implemented by professional staff or laypersons who work in any healthcare environment.

Hospital Arts programs have been successfully integrated into institutions in the United States and Europe. Reports in the *International Journal of Arts Medicine* (listed in Chapter 7) show that these programs relieve the boredom of patients, lift their spirits, and contribute to the healing process. The chapter on research covers some of the data that also show the cost-effectiveness of incorporating the arts into various units.

Preventive medicine is on the rise for several reasons: it cuts expenses and it is good for people who are ill or in recovery. The creative arts provide a simple, beautiful and noninvasive way to help people heal. When the community joins healthcare professionals, including creative arts therapists, the effort becomes a larger human enterprise of teamwork in the truest sense of the word. The Hospital Arts program at Utah Valley Regional Medical Center is the basis of the guidelines in each chapter of this manual. The program consists of 60+ volunteers, most of whom are music majors at Brigham Young University (BYU) who offer their talents as a service. The BYU program, directed by Professor Rosalie Rebollo Pratt, faculty advisor, and student directors who coordinate the volunteers in programs at the various facilities in the community, is supported by Art Access/Very Special Arts Utah, the Utah affiliate of the international organization Very Special Arts, a program of the Kennedy Center, Washington, DC. The guidelines offered in this manual have already been followed successfully in the Provo, Utah, community program. It is emphasized, however, that each community must create its own model based on the special needs of the people and facilities in the area. This guide will greatly assist in practical ways to get started. Chapter 8 of this manual describes three other hospital arts models that are among the most outstanding and effective in the world.

Grateful acknowledgment is hereby made of the caring artists who share their gifts with those whose health is compromised, and the generous nurses and physicians who have invited artists into their healthcare facilities. It is my hope that the basic ideas that have already succeeded in thriving, active Hospital Arts programs will inspire others to create their own programs and bring the gift of the arts back to the healing process.

Rosalie Rebollo Pratt
Provo, Utah, March 1997

CHAPTER 1

The Creative Arts in Healthcare: An Idea Whose Time Has Come

The hospital ward looked like any other, filled with uniformed persons hurrying among rooms, pushing poles with IV clear plastic bags, or marking charts at the nursing station. There were the usual visitors looking uneasily into rooms of semi-elevated beds with patients staring into tiny television sets suspended from the ceiling. Then I heard the sound of a cello playing the *Londonderry Air.* An attendant pushing a wheelchair patient back to her room paused at the door of the room from which the music was coming; the patient, who had signaled him to stop put her head forward to listen more closely to the melody. A smile crossed her face, she closed her eyes and began to nod in time to the rhythm. As the music continued, there were others who paused by the door, listened for a moment, smiled briefly, and then moved on.

I was in the ward that day as faculty advisor to a Hospital Arts program I began several years ago at Utah Valley Regional Medical Center in Provo, Utah. The idea was simple: invite young performers from our university to go into the hospital to play and sing for patients. They came with the tunes they knew, learned the songs and hymns the patients requested, and brought their gift of music to everyone in the hospital who cared to listen.

Since those early days the program has mushroomed to include several local healthcare facilities and retirement homes. Volunteers from the community have joined the students to bring music and other creative arts into the hospital environment. It is clearly an idea whose time has come. A new concept? Perhaps, to some. The linking of music and medicine, however, is as old as the earliest recorded accounts of healing. We know that Egyptian physicians used incantation for healing purposes, and the ancient Greeks also used chant, rhythm, and music to change mood and bring relief to patients with physical, emotional, and mental illnesses. The healing temples of the Egyptians and Greeks were havens for the sick and disabled; there they found mending of the body and spirit, since the priest/physician was able to bring harmony and restored order to both aspects of the human organism.

The shamans, medicine men and women, and healers of all kinds from medical traditions that have always lived side by side with orthodox techniques, never lost sight of the mind-body concept. Today, traditional medicine is looking to these healers whose frequently effective methods simultaneously address the patient's mental-emotional health and physical problems. Modern medicine is finally grasping the error of having separated the mind and body in healthcare. It is now clear that music (as well as the other creative arts) enhances well-being because it brings with it the order and balance that the Greeks understood when they spoke of a universal harmony of which man was a reflection. They knew that harmony within the body was related to a oneness with the universe, and a rhythmicity that exists in all living organisms. Current research in Germany and America is validating this concept as scientists actually witness and measure the rhythmicity in human organs and systems.

The reasons for reaching out to ancient traditions—those of the early Greeks as well as those of the contemporary nontraditional healer—are couched in the need to find simpler, more direct ways of facilitating healing. The expensive, and thereby exclusive, methods of high technology are so often out of the reach of the average patient that modern healthcare must now seek remedies for all patients that are simple and cost effective.

The miracle of putting music into healthcare is that it is so simple, yet so direct. Music touches everyone and is part of every human culture. Although most of us do relatively little to support any of the arts, it is impossible to think of daily life without music from our radios, our stereo players, the media, our schools, churches and synagogues, and places of business or pleasure. There is no formal mandate for music, yet we cannot live without it.

Anecdotal accounts from the earliest periods of western as well as eastern medicine attest to the use of music in healing. The earliest European universities dating back to the Middle Ages show the high place of music among the liberal arts. We know from student journals and lecture notes that these young people first learned the seven liberal arts of grammar, logic, rhetoric, astronomy, geometry, mathematics, and music. When, and only when, these seven arts were mastered could the student go on to the fields of theology, medicine, or the law. The earliest Greek medical writings speak of the need to understand musical principles in order to know how to take the human pulse. Galen wrote that the study of music was important in the education of the future physician. He spoke of Aesculapius, the son of Apollo, who composed melodies and in whose name healing temples were built. Apollo himself was god of medicine and music, and both Plato and Aristotle attested to the importance of music in the curriculum of the future leaders of the state. The writings of Greek physicians and philosophers clearly indicate that there was a very healthy respect for the effects of different musical modes, which could both incite or calm people's spirits and bodies. Flute music was said to help people digest their food after a heavy meal, and the appropriate music could drive away melancholy as well as calm a troubled spirit. It is important to understand that the Greek term for music included poetry and the spoken word. The arts in ancient Greece were far more connected than is the case in our time.

How then did music become separated from medicine? Actually, in practice it never did. Physicians throughout the Renaissance and Enlightenment continued to attest to the powers of music for healing persons who had experienced seizures, depressions, neurasthenia, and the like. It was even claimed that it could bring relief to persons who had been bitten by tarantulas. Although this last account has been challenged by Henry Sigerist as a hoax perpetrated by former pagans who needed a handy excuse to continue what would have been seen as inappropriate and outright sexual behavior by their new Christian guardians, the salubrious power of rhythmic movement is continually witnessed throughout history.

Descartes was the one who confused us most by separating the mind from the body. He told us that the mind was of one substance, the body of another, and thereby began our magnificent obsession with specialization. Since that time, university campus administrators and faculty have driven human knowledge into monastic cells called departments and isolated our intellectual inquiries from the contamination of other disciplines. All this has resulted in some admittedly spectacular high technology that somehow has distracted us from the fundamental fact that the human being is basically a network of living tissue and fluid directed by a wondrous brain that has always been receptive to suggestion—good or bad—and can actually cause all of the body systems to communicate with one another. The research of experts in a relatively new field called psychoneuroimmunology has awakened us to an intersystem networking about which we never dreamed.

Fortunately or unfortunately, depending on one's perspective, modern medicine has reached a crisis. We must find simpler, more direct ways to heal and in so doing we must begin to reclaim autonomy and responsibility for our own bodies and minds. Music in healthcare is a tool that can assist every person in that quest because it begins with the patient's choice. Once the patient has discovered the music that is "right", that is, the most healthful for him or her, the journey has begun. This music can then be used to help the person learn to relax, access inner resources of strength and calmness, and self-regulate. Self-regulation is an attitude toward health. It does not discount the wonderful advances of modern medicine, yet it first directs the patient toward a self-healing state of mind. The patient who is in control, calm, and relaxed will surely respond better to any medical intervention than a patient who is stressed, upset, and frightened. We now know that the immune system is affected directly by our frame of mind. Something as simple as S-IgA—the analysis of a saliva sample before and after an intervention to determine a measure of immunocompetence—can quickly illustrate the effects of music listening on patient well-being. The decrease in heart rate of a premature infant in an Intensive Care Unit, where a microcassette of lullabies has been placed in the isolette, graphically shows how the baby is calmed by the music. In every aspect of medical practice, music as well as the other creative arts can impact the well-being of patients in all stages of illness and recovery. Current music medicine research is confirming what we always knew, that the arts are fundamental to human health, and without them we are subject to unnecessary levels of stress, pain, and fear.

Until now we have seen pharmacology as the primary and immediate solution to these problems. Now, however, pharmacology is joined by the arts as handmaidens that help the patient reduce the need for outside interventions by accessing the inner wellsprings of health through the use of natural resources such as endorphins, the natural opiates of the body. Music is one of those natural remedies that is now often sought as a first method toward restoring patient well-being. The use of music and the other arts in healthcare facilities and private practices as well as institutions and private settings of all kinds is a dramatic new thrust in modern medicine. The techniques are simple, accessible, and, best of all, cost effective in a society in which healthcare reform must respond to this basic requirement.

It is important at this point to make some distinctions concerning the use of music in the healing environment. So far the discussion has been about bringing music into the healthcare environment. I would like to keep this separate from other uses of music in healing by referring to it simply as "music in healthcare". Music in healthcare includes professional as well as amateur musicians who usually volunteer their talents by playing or singing in healthcare facilities. It also includes such things as musicians who work with physicians to create audiotapes for office waiting rooms; or musicians who regularly bring music into retirement and nursing homes; or musicians who teach piano lessons to or sing songs with children in shelters; or musicians who regularly visit prison facilities or forensic units of hospitals to perform as well as teach small group instrumental classes. The musicians in these programs are trained musicians, artists of varying degrees of skill, often competent improvisers and accompanists. There is no claim made in these programs to directly provide a therapeutic intervention, something that requires specialized training. However there may be a therapeutic result as an outcome of these encounters with music.

Music in healthcare emphasizes music. The benefits that derive from these programs are due to the music and the artistry of the performer. Certainly there is also the human factor. Volunteers in these programs also perform a great service by making friends with the people to whom they bring their music.

Music therapy is a term that is sometimes used out of proper context to include any use of music for health-related purposes. A music therapist is a person who has been trained in an institution whose program is approved either by the American Music Therapy Association. A music therapist may become board certified by successfully passing a national examination. Music therapy programs differ among themselves in emphasis and rigor. Some music therapy programs produce graduates at the baccalaureate level, while others demand master's level competency. Music therapy, which actually developed following World War II from volunteer programs at veterans' hospitals, has become an important psychotherapy and has contributed significantly to human well being.

Special music education has contributed to human well-being by working in the educational arena with children who experience learning disorders. The emphasis here is on education, and understanding of pedagogy and learning styles is central to helping these children. The special music educator must often deal with groups of children who have a variety of learning as well as physical, emotional, and behavioral disorders. There are relatively few music educators trained in special education, just as there are relatively few special educators. The alarming incidence of learning disorders is forcing communities to look at new ways to help teachers cope with these problems.

MusicMedicine is probably the newest of all these terms. MusicMedicine is distinct in its direct and intentional link with the medical profession. This link is particularly emphasized in mutual research projects designed to help teams—often composed of musicians and physicians—to better understand the influence of music on all human behavior. Research projects that help us understand better how the brain and body are affected by musical stimuli also enlighten us about related medical, therapeutic, and educational matters. MusicMedicine also involves a branch of research that studies the phenomena associated with performance-related injury. It is not unusual to find MusicMedicine research teams today that involve the collaboration of a musician and a physician. Such models are effective because they bring together the knowledge, skills, and perspectives of two different yet closely related disciplines.

There are now hospitals, healthcare facilities, and private practices that include music and other creative arts as part of daily routine. The Utah Valley Regional Center Hospital Arts program, the Arts-in-Medicine program at Shands Hospital in Gainesville, Florida, the Medical Clinic III in Munich, and the Duke University Cultural Arts program are four good examples of productive arts-medicine models. As physicians and hospital personnel see the benefits of music medicine, the phenomenon grows and thrives. We have already entered a new era of healthcare and once again the words of Sir Francis Bacon speak eloquently to us:

> This variable composition of man's body hath made it as an Instrument easy to distemper; and therefore the Poets did well to conjoin Music and Medicine in Apollo, because the Office of Medicine is but to tune this curious Harp of man's body and to reduce it to Harmony.
> —Sir Francis Bacon. *The Advancement of Learning* Book 2. X. 1. 2.

CHAPTER 2

How to Incorporate the Creative Arts in a Hospital Environment

Getting started

Getting started is the hardest part of a Hospital Arts program. There are several excellent models described in detail in Chapter 8 of this manual. Reading about a program that is already well under way and highly successful can be intimidating to the novice. One might begin a new venture by identifying some modest immediate goals and then beginning a program by selecting a hospital both willing and accessible.

The Hospital Arts program in Provo, Utah, was begun by simply picking up a phone and calling Utah Valley Regional Medical Center. We spoke to one of the administrators who made an appointment for us to come in for a chat. Because of our affiliation with an academic institution, we brought along the Music Department Chair and several interested students. We were directed to a conference room where five or six staff members (including nurses and behavioral medicine personnel) joined us.

We began the meeting by pointing out that music is good for people and we would like a chance to regularly visit patients to sing and play for them. Some good person had already paved the way for this argument by having shown up often in the hospital, where he played harmonica solos to the delight of patients and staff. The administrator commented that patients as well as staff enjoyed the impromptu concerts, which were a welcome diversion in the daily routine.

The next part of the conversation dealt with specifics. We worked out ways for students to come to the hospital, get identification badges and devise a schedule for patients in the stroke unit. This seemed like the best place to start since there was a dining/recreation area with enough room for a small ensemble of musicians. The second step was to determine the best time to bring a small group to the unit. We decided on the 5:30 to 6:30 p.m. dining hour when patients were already assembled in the area.

The staff wanted to know what kinds of music we could offer patients. We talked about this and decided that simple folk tunes, hymns, and light classics would work best with a predominantly Christian population of patients who were in their 50s, 60s, and 70s. We also decided that the students needed to understand the general problems and issues involved with stroke patients as these affected expressive and receptive behaviors. Students also needed to understand basic hospital routine and etiquette so that they would not in any way interfere with them. Looking back at the history of the earliest music therapy programs, we were impressed with the fact that the first curricula in this discipline taught just such a course. In fact, what we now know as music therapy began with volunteers visiting World War II veterans convalescing in veterans' hospitals.

Our next step was to organize the student volunteers into small groups to visit the unit three times a week. We assigned each student to an evening that was relatively free for him or her. Next we asked one person per group to act as the coordinator and to give a lift to those volunteers who were without transportation. We set up a network so that each student was responsible for contacting a key person in the group if he or she could not come to the unit on a particular evening. Having begun with a relatively small and manageable group of students, it was easy to set up the mechanism for transportation. We also asked the coordinator to organize the program by asking each student in advance to prepare a short list of pieces that could be played on demand. Therefore, solos and ensembles pieces were arranged in a program that featured student performances and group participation on an evenly distributed basis.

Students were then given instructions by the hospital administration on the rules and policies of the hospital as they pertained to volunteers. They also received ID badges with their pictures and names and became versed in daily hospital protocol as well as the routines of hospital staff with whom they would have contact whenever they visited the unit. They learned to check in at the nurse's station of the unit to see if there were patients who needed a personal visit rather than a group experience. They gradually became sensitive to the needs of patients with specific physical and emotional problems.

The first visit was informal and the students presented a variety of short instrumental and vocal pieces. They had prepared several group participation songs and invited the patients to join in. Students who were not performing moved among the patients and sat near them, encouraging them to sing, clap, or tap in time to the music. The group coordinator took time to ask patients which songs they would like to hear during the next visit and made a list of the requests. At first, the patients were hesitant, due to two factors: they were unsure about this new experience; and many of them were suffering from some degree of speech impairment. By the third visit, patients were more ready to ask for specific songs and participate in group singing. Our small group of student-volunteers was launched and the Hospital Arts program was a reality.

To sum up the steps involved in setting up the initial program, the following suggestions are listed for instant reference:

Step 1. Assess your immediate goals and contact the nearest hospital that is willing and accessible. Keep the goals practical and realistic, and the agenda brief!

Step 2. Ask the hospital administrator to invite some key staff members to the first meeting. Ask specifically for floor nurses (your strongest allies), behavioral medicine staff, and interested doctors. Don't be discouraged if only a few staff members show up. Bring along some of the student volunteers.

Step 3. Begin by **briefly** describing the hospital arts program already in place at institutions throughout the country. Mention that the arts bring a degree of beauty and comfort to patients who have been temporarily separated from home and families. Mention also that experimental research has shown that the arts offer healing to the patients by reducing stress and anxiety levels. Describe to the staff some of the benefits reported in the research chapter of this manual and emphasize the value of the program to the different patient groups.

Step 4. Outline a simple program of a small group of volunteer musicians who could sing and play short favorite pieces for patients in a unit. Ask about an entity such as a stroke or rehabilitation unit that lends itself to a small group presentation in a place such as a dining area.

Step 5. Ask one of the volunteers to sing or play a brief and well-known piece that is also well-liked by the general community. Stay with a relatively quiet instrument or a gentle singing voice.

Step 6. Show that you and the group are aware of community and generation tastes by mentioning folk songs and hymns that are well-known and liked. (Allay their fears that the group plans on presenting an entire act of a Wagnerian opera!)

Step 7. Ask the hospital staff to tell you and volunteers about basic hospital protocol and to discuss any fears staff may have concerning a program such as this. Listen carefully and reassure the staff that the volunteers will work hard not to interfere with routines and will respect hospital policies.

Step 8. Ask the staff when volunteers could be briefed about basic hospital procedures and when they could obtain the necessary IDs before they make their first visit. Ask if it would be desirable to draw up a simple contract between the hospital and the program directors to be clear about expectations and policies. Make sure that all insurance issues are covered.

Step 9. Discuss the length of the first visit and finalize arrangements for volunteers, a piano, audio equipment if necessary, and any other needs. Try to keep everything simple and uncomplicated.

Step 10. Schedule a review meeting for the end of the first week of the program so that volunteers may receive feedback from administration and staff.

Above all, keep the tone of this meeting friendly and relaxed. Allay any fears that the program will disrupt hospital routine by keeping the discussion simple, to the point, and reassuring. Emphasize cooperation and the benefits to patient morale and happiness. Finally, go into the first hospital visit in as relaxed and friendly a manner as possible. This will reassure patients and staff and make them eager for a return visit—your most important short-term goal.

Putting Music and the Other Creative Arts throughout the Hospital

The Emergency Room (ER). The ER waiting room is one of the most stressful areas in the entire hospital because it is there that people imagine the worst scenarios. It is also where the creative arts can work their greatest power in distracting anxious people consumed with worry about the real and imagined.

Begin with the nurses and staff who run the unit. Discuss with them the benefits that the Hospital Arts program has provided for other units in the hospital. Artists and design specialists will have suggestions about making at least one part of this area a place of relaxation and soothing sound. For example, the waiting area of a wellness center we visited recently had a small waterfall that provided everyone there with a soothing peaceful sound that supported a quiet mood but did not intrude. Bring samples of audiotapes with music that is soft, melodic and uncomplicated. Examples of music that fits this description are provided in Chapter 7. Discuss making a master tape of this music that could be played at a low volume in at least one section of the area, leaving a segment of the room for those who want to watch television. Discuss ways in which healing murals could make the walls of the room more mindful of health and well-being. These are simple, nonintrusive and inexpensive ways to humanize the atmosphere of the area and provide a gentle aura of caring to people waiting for treatment or to hear about a loved one.

Recovery Areas and Other Waiting Areas. These are areas in which there is much boredom as families and individuals wait for news of patients, or patients themselves experience the first step of convalescence. Whatever the human situation, the same principles apply—people under stress need gentle and sustained comfort and support. In addition to the soft music, healing murals, and waterfall, think carefully about reading material for persons who are waiting long hours. Carefully selected books of poems, short stories, inspirational material that is general in nature, and other publications that are supportive and familiar to people from the community will be of far more value than out-of-date magazines about fishing, hunting, or movie stars. A sensitively arranged ambiance shows people that the hospital is a place where caring professionals have thought about providing support to patients and their families.

Always remember to take the time to make friends with floor nurses and those in charge of the various units. This will save a great many hours in the long run. If the administrators of a unit are on your side, you will be much more successful in implementing ideas to change existing environments and habits. Begin by emphasizing the benefits to patients and that happier patients make life easier for the staff. Have samples of your ideas for music tapes, pictures, or reading material. Stay with ideas that are simple and relatively easy to implement. The simpler the suggestion, the more likely it is to be accepted by the staff member.

Volunteer Resources. Draw on existing groups of artists, for example, students at a nearby college or university. Invite hospital personnel to share their talents. The Shands Arts in Medicine (AIM) program includes a band of physicians who perform Dixieland and other music for patients and staff. We know of at least two eminent physicians who are also professional clowns and love to show off their talents. The more the hospital staff members are involved in your efforts, the more receptive they will be to sustaining and even expanding the program.

Look to community members who have studied one or more of the creative arts. Strolling musicians, poets, puppeteers, mimes, clowns, dancers, actors are very welcome diversions to people who are forced to spend endless hours staring at hospital room walls and ceilings. It also gives these amateurs an opportunity to use their training in a way that satisfies them as performers. Again, do not start with too large a proposal. Work slowly to build your program, making sure at every juncture that you have provided coordinators with information about every new activity you begin. Keep in constant contact with floor personnel and administration so that you can act quickly on feedback, both positive and negative. Remind all your volunteers that they are bringing enjoyment to patients and to keep their presentations short, light, and nonintrusive.

Storytelling is a wonderful way to help pediatric patients forget that they are stuck in a room or ward rather than being out in the sunshine. This is a relatively simple activity that offers hours of enjoyment to children. Select someone who has a pleasant and clear speaking voice that is also well modulated. Find stories that are not too long and have interest for young minds, especially those that are in need of fantasy and diversion. Look for materials that include participation by the children, for example, the delightful *Gingerbread Man* story recorded on audiotape by the a cappella group *Pieces of Eight* (see Chapter 7).

Dancers have wonderful ways of reminding patients about the delight of human movement. These performers can scale down a presentation to fit the area of the room, yet still delight the patient with artistic movement. Watching a professional dancer can also inspire patients who need to use more physical movement to work harder at the exercises suggested by their physical therapists.

Whatever and whichever of the creative arts you incorporate in your program, keep it delightful, simple, and compatible with the hospital environment. The message of beauty and rhythm will soon be reflected in the faces of the patients. The arts by themselves have the benefit of reminding people in any health state that the aesthetic is what ultimately sustains us and makes up for the difficulties of life.

Audiotapes for Adult Patients Awaiting Surgery. In 1996, a pilot experiment in MusicMedicine research was carried out at the request of Nurse Marian North and her colleagues at Alta View Hospital in Sandy, Utah. The goal was to provide patients about to undergo a laparoscopy or arthroscopy procedure with music listening interventions before, during, and after surgery. A wide variety of audiotapes ranging from popular instrumental and country music to light classics was offered to these patients the night before scheduled surgery. Fifteen minutes before the procedure, the patient was given headphones and the tape of his or her choice to begin listening. The intervention continued during the procedure and 15 minutes into recovery room time. Surgeons, nurses, operating room staff, and patients noted that the patients who had the music listening intervention experienced significantly less need for postsurgical pain medication as compared with the patients who did not have this intervention. The surgeons decided to offer all surgical patients the same opportunity for music listening, and the insurance company that covers the hospital and many others in the state of Utah has also opted to make this intervention possible in the facilities in their group. It is clear that a simple tool such as music listening can make a difference in the comfort level of a surgical patient and may even diminish the need for pain medication.

Audiotapes for Children Awaiting Surgery. We are currently working with Primary Children's Hospital in Salt Lake City to create ways in which the arts can mitigate the sheer terror little children experience when they are about to undergo a surgical procedure. Depending on the nature of the surgery and hospital policies, the children may or may not be allowed to have their parents with them. Even when the child has visited the hospital and unit in advance and met the professionals involved in his or her operation, the actual moment of separation and movement into the operating theater is very stressful for a young person suddenly deprived of parental comfort and nearness and confronted with robed and masked people who are bending over the table and looking considerably formidable.

An audiotape prepared carefully in advance can offer the nearness of a mother's, father's, or sibling's voice to the child. Headphones can provide the sound transmission that should contain selected songs and short stories that are favorites of the child. The music and words can be interspersed with reassuring messages from Mom and/or Dad telling the child that they are very close by and it will all be over very soon. Give this suggestion well in advance to parents anticipating their child's surgery. Tell them this can be very simply made with an ordinary tape recorder and that background sounds of the family pet or the piano are also reassuring to the frightened child. The audiotape, prepared at a time when the parents are not under stress, will offer just the right support to the child.

Music in the Hospital Environment. For many years, the Sportkrankenhaus Hellersen, a hospital in Lüdenscheid, Germany has outfitted the rooms and waiting areas of the facility with stereo headphone sets. Patients are therefore able to avail themselves of music listening experiences during all periods of their hospital stay. This constitutes an investment on the part of the hospital, yet the astute administrator will soon realize the benefits of keeping patients content and occupied with music of their choice. The happily distracted patient is easier to work with and gives the healthcare givers the opportunity to focus on professional tasks. Nurses also report that patients listening to music of their choice are more amenable to taking their medications and completing the exercises or routines that are necessary for recovery.

Another area for music listening is in the outpatient or same-day surgical procedure units. Nurse Maureen Reilly reported in 1996 at the International Society for Music in Medicine Conference at University of Texas/San Antonio that patients undergoing cataract surgery were comforted by music listening during the procedures and that selected physiological outcome measures were positively affected. It is obvious that such interventions are helpful in several ways: the patient is distracted and comforted; the surgeon and staff can concentrate on the task at hand; a happier, less stressed patient will have a more positive impression of the surgeon and staff and the entire experience—a win-win situation. In addition, pain medications and pain perception are often reduced, again leading to the idea that one is better off in every way.

CHAPTER 3

The Creative Arts in a Private Practice

The Waiting Room

The Waiting Room of a private medical practice is often a place where a patient must spend as long as an hour or more to receive news about a diagnosis or the results of a test. During this time, patients may be bored, stressed, or both. Many waiting rooms provide a television, which may be diverting but also has these attendant problems: not everyone in the waiting room wants to see the same show; children do not want to see soap operas and adults are often weary of watching cartoons; and the news of the day may be stressful in itself.

In a private medical practice, the decor and materials offered to patients reflect the concern and thoughtfulness of the independent practitioner or physician group. Too often, people in a waiting room see an ambiance that has been put together without much thinking about patient needs. Perhaps this is a new practice and the physician or physicians have simply taken over another person's ideas. Understandably, the practitioner is preoccupied with matters of the practice itself and matters of decor are left up to a receptionist or a wife who is also beset with the problems of settling her family into a new home and getting children ready for school. As a result, the old pictures, color scheme, wall paint, and furniture are left in place. Perhaps photographs of the doctor's family are mounted on the walls, and ancient copies of magazines that have little or nothing to do with patient comfort are strewn about the tables.

Waiting Room A. Imagine sitting in a physician's outer office, concerned about an impending diagnosis or treatment, and finding yourself in a shabby chair upholstered in a bright orange, looking at walls that are painted in a drab beige, peering at year-old magazines about fishing, and glancing up to sniff some stale coffee coming from an urn that was started 5 hours earlier. A television set is blaring news about a new skirmish in the Middle East and children with nothing to do are squabbling in a corner.

Waiting Room B. Now imagine the same office with a new coat of soft pastel paint, a small water cascade in the center of the area, the aroma of a lemon- or almond-scented potpourri, and some healing murals with messages of joy and life affirmation. Your chair is a soft brown fabric and nearby there are copies of magazines and pamphlets about healing. In the background there is soft music of a gentle rhythm and conjunct melodic nature, unintrusive yet comforting. There is a children's corner with quiet but interesting toys to play with. The atmosphere is reassuring and supportive.

In which waiting room would you rather be? How much time, effort, and resource did it take to make the changes from Waiting Room A to Waiting Room B? The difference in Waiting Room B gives the patient one clear message—this healthcare giver is concerned about me and my needs. He or she is thinking about my feelings and comfort and has given me a place to wait that indicates I will receive the same kind of attention and regard when I am undergoing treatment.

Instead of offering Waiting Room A as the only alternative, go into your outer office and try to imagine incorporating some of the following suggestions:

1. Look critically at the color on the walls. Is it restful? Think of some gentle colors that might soften the general look of the room. Ask a friend or colleague who has an artistic eye to give suggestions about colors that will fit a general scheme of rest and relaxation. The accent is on the collective appearance of the room, including wall color, furniture, fabrics, accents, reading materials, floor covering, and the like.

2. Examine the pictures or wall hangings in the office. Large pictures of your children may be very beautiful, but what comfort do they offer your patients, who may not even know these youngsters? Perhaps these family portraits are more suitable in your inner or private office where you might share with a patient some parental pride about your family. Instead consider displaying in your waiting room healing murals or landscapes that are filled with gentle rhythmic movement of color and space. Stay away from the overpowering picture and look for the piece that suggests tranquillity and invites the viewer inside. Rhythm is the basis of all life. There are many healthcare environments in the world that now pay special attention to wall hangings and their effect on patient well-being. Investigate some of these ideas and again consult your colleagues with expertise in artistic matters.

3. Offer some kind of peaceful but nonintrusive sound, such as falling water. Place this sound source in a central location of the room so that patients have a choice of being close or distancing themselves somewhat.

4. Look at the design and fabrics of the chairs in the room. Are they comfortable, soft, pleasant? Look at the formation of chairs in the area. Do the various seating arrangements suggest different groupings? Or are they all lined up against a wall? Consider the placement of small but attractive live plants among the various seating arrangements.

5. Check the reading material in your office. Do you have considerable variety in age-appropriate books and other publications? Story books for children with beautiful color illustrations can be very helpful toward distracting a tired, bored little boy or girl. Do you have quiet but clever activities that also help children while away the time? For the adults, select carefully chosen short stories, inspirational material, and don't forget publications that help people take responsibility for their own well-being. Take the time to go with members of your office staff to a bookstore where you can choose appropriate reading material. Investigate magazines and journals that help people understand the

connections between mind and body and how the arts can facilitate this. For example, a magazine such as *Common Boundary* offers informative and well written articles about healing. The *International Journal of Arts Medicine* includes excellent articles about the creative arts in healing. Look in Chapter 7 for other suggestions.

6. Offer your own suggestions in a brochure or newsletter. Include ideas about deep abdominal breathing (which helps patients calm down and access their parasympathetic systems) and autogenics. If you can spare an office worker, have him or her come into the waiting room every hour or so and lead the group in simple relaxation exercises. This accomplishes two purposes: the patients will be in a less stressed condition when they reach you; and they will become aware that this is a wellness office where the professional staff care about their well-being. A personal written message from the physician can go far to assure a patient that he or she is important to the practitioner. Something as brief as "We will do everything in our power to make your visit and treatment with us as comfortable and pleasant as possible. Please let us know what we can do to help you feel at ease and welcome" is wonderful reassurance to a patient.

7. If possible, ask a professional biofeedback provider to visit your office and train your staff in simple relaxation techniques. If you and your staff members understand how to relax even in the middle of a very busy day, that sense of calmness will spill over to the patients. Better yet, if you have a biofeedback provider in your community ask that person to provide biofeedback sessions for individual patients who are particularly stressed or in pain. Biofeedback is a way of using electronic instruments to help a person receive information about such functions as muscle tension, peripheral skin temperature, and skin resistance. As the person learns to control or manipulate the instrumental signal he or she gains control of the bodily response to some degree. Biofeedback is no longer experimental and it is clear that the more a person understands how to self-regulate, the better he or she can cope with physical or emotional illness. Join hands with your biofeedback provider. You will soon see the benefits in empowered patients. Contact the Association for Applied Psychophysiology and Biofeedback in Wheat Ridge, Colorado for more information.

> Association for Applied Psychophysiology and Biofeedback
> 10200 W. 44th Ave., Suite 304
> Wheat Ridge, CO 80033-2840
> (303) 422-8436

8. Show the members of your own staff that you understand the importance of preventive medicine. Invite a biofeedback provider to visit your office one morning before patients arrive. Let the provider give you and the staff a demonstration of how biofeedback techniques help people to understand control of autonomic system functions. In this age of escalating healthcare costs, you can be a powerful leader in helping healthcare professionals as well as patients understand the importance of gaining control of autonomic system func-

tions. Please see Chapter 6 for some research summaries of studies that show the power of biofeedback techniques with women in childbirth, performance majors, and children with attention deficit disorder or other learning disabilities.

9. Take the time to have regular sessions with your office staff to discuss human concerns as well as the details of the practice. How are all of you meeting patient needs and comfort? How can the practice develop ways to reassure and provide simple hospitality for patients? What are some ways in which we can let patients see our concern, such as providing a basket of fresh fruit every day, the personal message, the way in which the patient is greeted? Do we simply ask for demographic data or completion of forms? Or are we also giving our patients the idea that we are genuinely concerned with their comfort and well-being?

Healthcare is changing dramatically and physicians are quickly learning that they must provide more personal touches in order to attract and keep patients. Health management systems have changed the way care is given and the ways in which patients perceive their healthcare. The physician is now more accountable for his or her personal approach to a patient and the manner in which treatment is administered. In many ways this has been a good change because it helps physician and patient become partners in seeking wellness and homeostasis. We are seeing less and less of the aloof doctor in a starched white coat and more of the concerned healer who wants to work with a patient to achieve the best possible results in the most effective manner.

I remember a physician who invited me to speak to a morning office session with his staff. I was asked to talk about incorporating music and graphic arts into the practice and I came prepared to address a group of professionals about whose level of interest I was uncertain. I was pleasantly surprised to meet a staff of people who were obviously at ease with each other, were genuinely concerned about improvements to the practice, and talked about patients as real people. It was clear that this was a practice run by a physician who had imparted a sense of caring and concern for every person who sought help at his hands. The friendliness of the staff spilled over into the general environment of the office, which was softly decorated and inviting in every aspect. I remember leaving the facility thinking that this was one family practitioner I would remember with respect and a very pleasant recollection.

The best time to address issues concerning office environment is at the beginning of a practice. This sets the tone for everything that follows and for patients' first and lasting impressions of their caregiver. However, it is always appropriate to make needed changes and people will always respond to the physician who shows that he or she is looking first and foremost for patient well-being.

CHAPTER 4

Music and the Other Creative Arts for the Elderly

Music and the creative arts are vital for the well-being of older people. At this time in life, when physical and mental faculties become influenced by normal and abnormal effects of the aging process, the arts can stimulate, focus, and encourage activity. One of the immediate losses attendant to age is the inability to drive a car. Without a vehicle, the older person is automatically distanced from daily interaction with community members. Casual shopping, conducting business transactions, dining out, going to the bank are now activities that must be planned well in advance and organized so that they may all be taken care of at the same time, when the elderly person has access to transportation.

The resultant trouble and inconvenience tend to make the elderly person withdraw, stay at home, and turn to the television set for some kind of human input. Daily chores and needs such as taking out the garbage, doing minor household repairs, and even food shopping eventually become so fraught with dangers of slipping or, worse, falling, that the elderly tend to choose a retirement home community or, if their health warrants it, a nursing home. In many cases, this is the best solution for all concerned, especially for members of the extended family whose own familial responsibilities or jobs keep them from providing the necessary care for a relative. With concern for rising healthcare costs and cuts made to programs for the elderly, it becomes more pressing to find ways to enhance good health and well-being.

Setting Up the Program

Modern nursing homes and retirement homes are becoming more conscious of and sensitive to the emotional needs of the elderly. Cut off on a regular basis from events such as concerts, movies, theater, and other entertainment, these older people are the delighted recipients of the services of musicians and artists who take the time to bring the arts into their environment.

One of the greatest benefits of this arrangement is to bring music majors and older people together. The young student needs an audience for music to be performed in a senior or graduate recital; the older person loves to hear live performances of songs, piano sonatas, and ensemble pieces that bring back memories of concert-going days. The students in the Brigham Young University (BYU) Hospital Arts program are thrilled with the unconditional enthusiasm they receive when they perform recital pieces. Older ears are far more forgiving than faculty juries, and they are probably much more genuinely appreciative of the performance.

Before you make your first visit to the facility, contact the home supervisor—often a husband and wife team. Discuss the needs and backgrounds of the people in the facility and work out visitation schedules that include group performances as well as individual recitals. There are certain adjustments to be made for presenting recitals. Choose program coordinators who have an interest in elderly populations or have experience with an older relative.

The following suggestions are offered to help prepare programs appropriate for facilities designed for middle class residents, many of whom are retired professionals and their spouses:

1. Choose repertoire that is basically familiar to the audience, that is, music from the Baroque, Classical, Romantic, and Impressionistic periods.

2. Keep the entire recital within a reasonable listening period for people who cannot sustain a sitting position for very long; 45 minutes is probably just right, even 30 minutes may be more appropriate.

3. Use a microphone for announcements and for singers. Remember that many people in the audience have hearing loss.

4. Before each piece, tell the audience something brief and interesting about the work and place it in a time period for them. Remember that brief and interesting are the operative terms.

5. After the recital be sure to go among the members of the audience and get to know them. You will be amazed to find the variety of professions and backgrounds. Our first chats with retirement home people turned up doctors, lawyers, a judge, and a nationally known architect. There were people who spoke with great emotion of the pleasure they experienced in hearing a song or a sonata movement that was familiar.

6. Ask for names of favorite composers. Share students' repertoire with residents and respond to their preferences for certain pieces. Tell personal stories of developing as musicians and experiences with recitals and other performances. Make it a truly personal experience.

7. Schedule a feedback session with the residence directors or supervisor and listen carefully. Adjust dates and times of visits and keep learning about the needs of your audience.

8. Prepare well in advance for special religious and secular holidays. Our biggest eye-opener was that our holiday programs were often IT for some of the residents whose families who could not visit them. Be sure to include group singing and participation at holiday time. Carol singing, for example, can be a very important activity for these people. We have often noticed how residents dress up in their fanciest clothes for our visits at holiday time. The red dresses and dark suits suddenly appear because we have provided an occasion for looking particularly nice. Also bear in mind that dressing up and looking one's best are positive indications of healthy behavior.

9. Do not disappoint your audience. Impress on the performers that their visits are often the highlight of the week and substitutes must be found when a scheduled artist cannot be present.

10. Older people tend to be direct, sometimes blunt, in their comments. Our students have learned to become accustomed to comments about preferred pieces or performances that were judged to be better than others. Older people are very much like very young people—they say what is on their minds.

Setting up Resident Groups

Active participation can be encouraged among older people by organizing groups of singers into choirs and simple instrumental ensembles. We have witnessed very enthusiastic choirs and one of the local retirement homes has its own rhythm band, which consists of simple rhythm instruments that are played along with a student band or small ensemble. The resident band was so enthusiastic that they even made uniform vests to identify themselves as a group. The pièce de résistance came when they went "on tour" to other retirement and nursing homes in the community. Among other benefits, it gave these people a sense of contribution.

Remember that these resident groups are for fun. Encourage vigorous participation, but keep activities at a level where enjoyment rather than hard work is the motto. Choose singing and instrumental music that is suitable. If you have someone who is an old clarinet player and would like to try his or her hand at that again, encourage this by all means. Revive old interests in a high school or college instrument, if the desire is there. Give players parts that are simple yet interesting. Do not concern yourself with unusual instrumentation. You may have something as exotic as several maracas, a violin, a kazoo, and some hand drums. Who cares! Just make music and let the sound take care of itself. The process, not the product, is the important outcome.

Recruiting Community Volunteers

When United Way listed our Hospital Arts program in their brochures, we began to hear from community members, including church groups, high school students, and amateur artists. Involving these community members forges a link among people and generations. Teenagers need opportunities to learn firsthand about special needs populations. Including them in Hospital Arts programs teaches them patience, compassion, and respect for others far better than lectures and threats. They will never find more generous or appreciative listeners than older people in retirement homes and nursing facilities. They will also learn music other than the kind they listen to regularly, and in so doing will expand their understanding of repertoire and styles. The bonding that comes between a teenager and an older person through the arts is a lasting link that enriches both. As always, educate the young performer ahead of time as to appropriate selections and performance mode.

Church choirs and other community groups are often very eager to perform and appreciate the opportunities to share their talents. In addition to these ensembles, seek out the semiretired singer, pianist, harpist, flutist who has been putting most of his or her effort into another primary occupation such as home-making or a career in business. Don't neglect to invite the staff of the home or nursing facility to join in, and above all do not forget your physicians and nurses, many of whom are ardent amateur musicians and long for a chance to perform.

Careful advertising of the Hospital Arts program will attract many people from groups such as those described above. As always, apprise all performers of the rules and policies of the institution and make sure they understand the needs and preferences of the people for whom they will perform. Attention to these details will ensure a joyous and productive experience for all involved.

One of the greatest human benefits of the program will be the interpersonal contacts among the residents and the performers. As the performers come to know the residents personally, they will begin to ask about people and matters of importance to their new friends. Performing for someone you know and care about brings about a certain satisfaction that is absent from a presentation to strangers. As with all other segments of a Hospital Arts program, look for feedback and listen carefully for suggestions to improve or adjust the presentations. Our experience has been that residents ask for more recitals and ensemble programs, particularly around holiday time. This, of course, will vary from place to place. Keep track of the learning experiences of your performers and use them to improve the program from year to year. Our performers are asked to keep a journal in which they record their notes about each visit.

Impress upon the young performers that this is among the humanly important aspects of sharing their art. Help them understand that audiences do not exist only in concert halls but that there is a rich and vast group of listeners eager to respond to art in every form. For many residents of nursing and retirement homes, the music that is brought to them through Hospital Arts programs is the only live music that will consistently appear in the remainder of their lives. We have often heard our BYU performers comment on the warm responses and generous applause they receive from older listeners. This can be sharing art at its most important and humanly significant level and it can also help young people to understand the value of reaching out to a segment of society they are seldom encouraged to even notice.

CHAPTER 5

People in Crisis or Difficult Circumstances

The Hospital Arts program in Provo, Utah, has helped us realize the extent of human suffering in a single community. Some of this pain cannot be helped; much of it, however, is preventable. Violence and depressed economies are often significant factors in some of the groups we visit. Although the causes of the problems are far-reaching, and solutions are beyond the grasp and purview of this volume, there is always the considerable joy and comfort that comes to many of these people through the arts. In this chapter, we will describe some facilities and groups who can benefit from the services of a Hospital Arts program.

Family Support and Crisis Centers

Centers for Women and children in crisis are appearing in all communities. These facilities provide immediate shelter and respite from abusive or potentially abusive situations. Here we find children in residence for as little as a few hours or as much as a week or more. House parents, approved after very careful screening by the licensed supervisors, are the surrogate guardians who attend to the children's needs. Many of these centers have to deal with a rotating schedule of house parents, a factor that may increase the anxiety of a child who is already stressed. Sometimes a child may be dropped off very suddenly by a parent who knows he or she is getting out of control. Children in this situation often exhibit withdrawal behavior, which is understandable when one considers the circumstances of being placed in the center.

The Hospital Arts program can perform a number of services. Since contact will often be with children, suggestions will be made primarily with youngsters in mind. Begin by assessing the general setup. Is there a room large enough for some movement activities and song games? We found a donor who presented a center with a used upright piano that worked very well for our needs. Audiotapes work well for musical accompaniment to activities, stories, and background music for other quiet-time work such as coloring or drawing. Some of our more creative volunteers even set up a beginning piano lesson program that introduced the instrument to children who were interested. Group singing also helps create a dynamic atmosphere that can then lead to other activities.

Help volunteers learn a repertoire of songs that are fun to sing and invite participation. Do not press a child to join in. Many of these children have been very disappointed by adults and are reticent to invite a relationship with a stranger. Always let the children know that they are welcome at any time to join a group or just watch if they wish.

Sometimes children in crisis will want to talk as they become involved in an activity that helps them relax. Volunteers should be trained to listen, not to prod, and to let the child know that if any subject of abuse, violence, or witnessed criminal behavior is addressed, that the volunteer is obliged to report that to the program director. It is inappropriate for volunteers to initiate discussions about the reasons for the children being in the center. Emphasize the need to keep promises. Always try to keep a scheduled visit. You are often working with a child who has known a life full of broken promises—he or she does not need another one.

It is amazing to recall the many positive experiences in centers. Even though the children come and go, there is a lingering gift of the art that has been brought to their midst, if only for a day. Diversify the activities to include children ranging in age from preschool to upper elementary. Bring simple rhythm instruments, or help children make them from scratch.

Shakers. You can make simple shakers from small one-serving milk cartons. Empty the carton, rinse, and dry thoroughly. Next, fill it with rice or small beans. Close the lid and you have a very effective shaker.

Drums. Simple drums can be made from discarded coffee cans (retain the plastic lid), oatmeal cartons, or any kind of medium size cylindrical container. These can be decorated with construction paper and colored with the children's art work.

Sticks. Ask a carpenter for some discarded dowels. Trim these down to size and you have rhythm sticks, which can also be painted with bright colors (nonlead paint, please!).

Jingle Bells. We have made some very lovely jingle bells from items found in novelty or notion departments. These can be strung together as wristlets or anklets and provide beautiful tinkling accompaniment to many songs.

The Severely Developmentally Disabled

Facilities for the Severely Developmentally Disabled are places where music can often bring some degree of response, even if it is not always apparent. Creative Arts Therapists have made wonderful contributions to these facilities and music performers can enhance their work. Again, assess the situation and ascertain which units could most benefit from some live music. If there is a music therapist on staff, consult with her to program music she feels will most benefit the patients. Unfortunately, budget cutbacks in these institutions have often deprived them of the services of creative arts therapists, and you will probably have to work with a staff member who is more in the line of an occupational therapist. Be sure that you go over with staff members the kind of music that your group can offer and discuss how stimulative or sedative it needs to be—a very important factor among these populations. Then plan the kinds of music to be offered according to the guidelines suggested by the staff. Remember that they know the patients and their reactions best.

Once the program coordinator has worked out a plan for the first event, carefully instruct all volunteers about the institution's policies and how the program fits into existing routines. Discuss the populations the volunteers will come into contact with and prepare them to accept any appropriate response, as small as it may be. Most of them will not at first understand why there may be little recognition from residents.

Participation should be on a basis that accommodates the functional level of the residents. Some residents—with some creative help—can participate with rhythm instruments. We know of an ingenious musician who has worked out systems for taping sticks and bells to the wrist to help people with little function handle the instrument. Your music or occupational therapist can be of great assistance in this matter. Always encourage participation but never press too hard. Offer the activity and invite people to join in. Notice the comfortable level of functioning and try to stay within that boundary to help the person enjoy the music and not be frustrated by a process that is too difficult.

Bring audiotapes of music and give suggestions to the staff for a variety of recorded pieces that can be played on the P.A. system during mealtime or other periods of the day. Try to recruit local artists to offer suggestions for healing murals and other kinds of visual stimuli. Dancers can offer aesthetic stimulation through demonstrating simple movements in response to music. Research has clearly shown that movement in response to auditory stimuli contributes to enhanced motor function. All of these activities, however, must first be cleared with the appropriate staff in order to ensure the safety of residents and adherence to institutional policies.

Forensic Units

Particular caution must be exercised with populations in hospital units for residents who have exhibited criminal behavior. Our experience shows that volunteers must always go in groups. Before they start, they must be thoroughly briefed by the appropriate staff member about the strict rules and policies of the unit. There is little chance of an unfortunate incident as long as volunteers understand and adhere to rules, stay in groups, and are always sure that there are sufficient numbers of hospital technicians during the actual program presentation. Some basic rules include:

1. Do not give patients your last name or any other personal information such as your phone number.

2. Avoid all body contact, even hand shaking.

3. Do not take any messages from patients or offer to communicate with anyone on the outside.

4. Keep the program a mix of solo, ensemble, and group participation. Photocopy words of songs and have them ready to give the patients before you begin each program.

5. Make sure that there is a mature person who is acting as the program coordinator who will watch especially for adherence to all policies, especially maintaining proper distance from the patients.

6. Some units will actually want to include hymns in the group singing. In other cases, this will not be an appropriate type of music. Here is an instance where feedback is crucial.

7. Carefully check on all insurance matters. These units often have blanket policies. If volunteers are from an educational institution, clear the program with college or university administration.

8. Be candid with volunteers about not being drawn toward any kind of emotional involvement with the residents of the unit. Misguided empathy or sympathy may lead to a very unfortunate situation. It is because of this point that we particularly stress the need for a mature and assertive coordinator.

In all of our experience, we have avoided any unpleasant experiences, even when some of the patients in the room were convicted murderers and violent people. Careful observance of the rules mentioned above has made this a very rewarding part of the program, and we have witnessed as much gratitude and appreciation for our visits in a forensic unit as we have seen from any other group in the entire program.

Homeless Abuse Victims Shelters

Unfortunately for society, shelters for homeless and abuse victims are becoming a fact in most communities. Here, as in the crisis centers, the arts can especially serve the children. Those who have lost their own homes and rooms are greatly in need of something that reminds them of security and support systems. Bring songs that are familiar, cheerful, and have activities. Follow the guidelines for the instrument and movement activities suggested above. Determine the actual space you will have to work in and gear activities toward the area size. Here again, you will be dealing with transient populations. Stick with simple, catchy songs that are easy to learn or relearn.

There are also adults who need the benefit of the arts. Again, choose repertoire that is familiar and easily put together. Group participation often offers a catharsis to stressed adults who have little opportunity for expression under circumstances that are very difficult.

Wherever possible, recruit storytellers, puppeteers, mimes, and, if you are fortunate to have them among you, poets. For many people in crisis, nonverbal expression is easiest and most desirable; for others, the chance to express feelings in poems and short essays or stories is fulfilling. All this can be determined by the needs of the people in the facility and your own resources.

General Guidelines for All Special Populations

1. Carefully assess the unit and facility and match your resources with possibilities offered by available space and time. Appoint a strong, mature, assertive program coordinator.

2. Thoroughly discuss your program with the unit or institutional administrators and staff. Offer several kinds of activities and ask for candid feedback.

3. Investigate the rules and policies of the institution, including all matters pertaining to insurance coverage. In this situation, it is important to have a document in writing that clearly sets out the expectations and responsibilities of the facility and the Hospital Arts volunteers.

4. Instruct all volunteers prior to the first visit about the populations they will be serving, the policies of the institution or unit, and the specific rules they must observe. Obtain ID badges for volunteers so that they are properly identified at all times when they are in the facility.

5. Instruct the program coordinator to obtain regular feedback on the program from unit or institutional personnel and residents. This will help greatly in appropriately modifying the presentations.

6. Whenever possible, invite residents to participate. Involvement in an artistic activity is in itself positive action.

CHAPTER 6

Fund Raising and Research

Budget

The good news is that Hospital Arts programs are relatively inexpensive. Since the program largely depends on volunteer artists, costs are reduced to administration, equipment, supplies, and advertising. These can be kept at very modest levels. The BYU program has managed to get along well on volunteers and support from Art Access/Very Special Arts Utah, the Utah affiliate of the international organization Very Special Arts, a program of the Kennedy Center, Washington, DC. The faculty director of the program donates her services, and the student director and her assistants are allotted a modest yearly amount to cover their time in coordinating activities and volunteers. The rest of the budget is spent on music, disposable supplies, activities, brochures, and selective advertising. Based on an annual budget of about $1500, funds are usually allocated as follows:

Administration	35%
Supplies	15%
Activities	35%
Brochures	15%

This allocation varies with the yearly plans. It gives us, however, a good idea of basic funds distribution. In a period in which accountability is more and more important, detailed receipts and accounts must be kept to be presented at the year's end to the funding organizations. Your coordinators, directors and assistants need to follow a plan for obtaining prior permission for any expenditures and then keeping receipts that are turned over to the person in charge of accounts. The simpler the program, the easier it is to keep all of this straight. We have our money in a separate account so that there is no problem with confusion of funds from other projects. Simplicity and a straightforward system that is easy to manage and report should be your guide. The more elaborate the system the more time it will take to prepare for an end-of-the-year audit.

Our program is also enriched by donations, such as the piano that was contributed to a family crisis center. As your program becomes more established, donors of instruments and artistic items will start to appear. You will soon find that these donations are very important to the program.

United Way has listed us in their roster of community services and programs and other community organizations have called to inquire about our work. We always ask established and reputable organizations to list us, because this is effective and free advertising.

Research

Our Hospital Arts program is part of a larger effort known as MusicMedicine. MusicMedicine is a field that has evolved in the 90s as a result of exploration of links to several disciplines. MusicMedicine focuses on a very close relationship with the field of medicine and encompasses all aspects of music and the healing process, including: (a) effects of music on selected physiological aspects of human behavior and function; (b) music and psychotherapy; (c) music and bio- and neurofeedback; (d) music and specific clinical applications such as pre-, peri-, and postoperative surgical procedures; (e) music and educational issues for special populations; and (f) music and performance-related injuries. In concept and execution, MusicMedicine is based on strictly controlled experimental research and, because of this, theoretical knowledge in the area of effects of music on physical, emotional, and mental behavior is gaining ground as well as acceptance in the scientific community.

Music Therapy and MusicMedicine have contributed substantially to the progress of behavioral medicine and healthcare. Since the 1950s, Music Therapy has been the oldest pioneer in bringing the influence of music to bear in virtually every aspect of medical practice. Music Therapy is involved in many of the activities described above and has developed an important position in modern healthcare. Training programs vary in clinical or theoretical emphasis; degrees are granted at both the baccalaureate and master's levels; and, although current research is becoming more rigorous in design and implementation, many studies in the literature are based on anecdotal and case history reports. Music Therapy has evolved into a field that offers the practitioner an excellent venue for practice in institutions, small or large groups, or private practice on a one-on-one basis. The professional directories in the field illustrate the vast breadth of specialties available to the future music therapist. Music therapists often work in teams with other healthcare professionals and, depending on the part of the country or globe, their services are in different degrees of demand.

MusicMedicine, on the other hand, has from the beginning made a direct effort to keep training and research at the graduate level and is unquestionably allied in all its activities with the medical profession. MusicMedicine also attracts a variety of interested and qualified professionals in symposia and conferences, including educators, musicians, physicians, psychologists, nurses, and others in the allied health fields. The inclusionary aspect of MusicMedicine enriches the research product, since musicians and physicians join hands in projects, thereby broadening the dialogue and scope of the design and protocol. MusicMedicine seems to have entered the arena of interdisciplinary healthcare with ease, perhaps because of its very inclusionary position. The objective is to produce hard, objective, and defensible research that will be respected by the larger scientific community. In this effort, musicians from different backgrounds of professional emphasis are fitting comfortably into a field that clearly bases its strength on the knowledge and insights of many disciplines. As a field, MusicMedicine is quite new and the role of the researcher/practitioner is still being defined. A Ph.D.

program in MusicMedicine as a peer specialty in behavioral medicine has already been proposed (see Pratt & Spintge, 1996, *MusicMedicine,* volume 2, St. Louis: MMB Music).

Biofeedback, Neurofeedback, and MusicMedicine Research: BYU Program
In 1990, the author began a master of arts degree program at Brigham Young University. Thesis studies under the direction of Pratt and colleagues in medicine as well as the arts have developed into a series of projects that illustrate the benefits of music in the healthcare environment. These studies have included the following projects (please see Selected References section for complete bibliographic information):

1. The Effects of Music and Biofeedback on Stress Reduction of Music Majors (Niemann, Pratt, & Maughan, 1994).
2. The Effects of Live Music on Selected Physiological Measures of Recovering Heart Surgery Patients (Weber, unpublished master's thesis, 1994).
3. The Effects of Selected Music Listening and Biofeedback on Cardiac Chronotropic Control of Women in Childbirth (Lex, Pratt, Abel, & Spintge, 1995).
4. The Effects of Selected Music Listening on S-IgA Levels of Patients Undergoing Crown Replacement (Goff, 1995, unpublished master's thesis).
5. The Effects of Background Music on Neurofeedback Training of Children with Attention Deficit Disorder (Pratt & Abel, 1995).
6. The Effects of Female and Male Singing and Speaking Voices on Selected Physiological Measures of Premature Infants in an Intensive Care Unit (Coleman, Pratt, Stoddard, & Abel).

These studies have yielded important information that is presently being disseminated among interested physicians and healthcare facilities, including hospitals and medical centers. The most important news to the healthcare community is that our studies indicate the cost-effective benefits of music listening.

In the most highly controlled circumstances, we have shown that premature infants (n = 33) who listen to a minimal amount of recorded female and male singing on microcassettes in their isolettes gain significantly more weight during the intervention period, take in more calories and leave the unit an average of just under 3 days earlier than carefully matched control infants. At a possible cost of thousands of dollars per infant per day in the unit, the savings to the hospital can be significant.

The S-IgA study shows that female patients respond with greater immunocompetence to selected music listening than they do to nitrous oxide. This is especially important to dentists who cannot administer nitrous oxide to pregnant female patients. The difference between the significant positive female response and the less positive male response to the music intervention raises an important question. Is this a biological brain difference between the sexes and, if so, why did it not show up with the premature infants?

The study with the ADD children showed that those who received neurofeedback training and background music (Mozart) scored in the 20th percentile (median) as compared to the control group (without music) who scored in the 9th percentile (median). These results are from the *McCarney Test* (Home Version). Six months following the neurofeedback intervention, 70% of the children are still maintaining focus and concentration in their schoolwork. Neurofeedback is especially important for children with ADD who do not respond to or cannot tolerate drugs usually prescribed for the disorder.

Biofeedback, especially biofeedback training with selected music listening, benefits women in childbirth. In another highly controlled study, women with both interventions achieved greater heart rate variability and decreased heart rate during labor at 4 cm dilation. Eight of nine primiparas opted for music listening only during labor and did not request epidurals. Biofeedback and music listening were also effective in diminishing reported stress of music performance majors pre- and posttested at jury time. The study with recovering heart patients showed a trend toward increased peripheral skin temperature following 15 minutes of live music performance.

A recent study of sexually molested children with Attention Deficit Disorder (ADD) using EEG Neurofeedback and music listening has indicated that music also works as an enhancer of the neurofeedback training process. Children in this program are additionally challenged with the serious effects of sexual molestation and it is vital that our training program works in strict lockstep with the ongoing therapy program for the child. Our research is presently being conducted with the Family and Attachment Center in Salt Lake City, Utah. Initial studies show that the EEG neurofeedback training and background music listening are helping children with ADD who have experienced the tragedy of sexual molestation to regain focus and control over negative behaviors associated with Attention Deficit Disorder.

Another study in neurofeedback training and music listening involves female subjects with Chronic Fatigue Immune Dysfunction Syndrome (CFIDS). Preliminary work has shown the positive effects of this intervention toward relieving fibromyalgia, one of the more debilitating aspects of CFIDS.

All of the above studies are a beginning, but an important solid step toward controlled defensible evidence of the effects of music on the human life process. Music Medicine Associates Research Group (MMARG) will continue to conduct and monitor research in this area. The collaboration of a music educator and physician provides a rich linkage between the two professions and much greater insight into the phenomena being observed.

Research in MusicMedicine or any kind of Arts Medicine must follow these rules:

1. Choose a significant and timely, relevant topic for investigation and create a research design that is carefully controlled and will yield objective data.

2. Seek funding from science foundations as well as service groups, corporations, and the like.

3. Involve artists and healthcare professionals. Physicians and nurses are excellent collaborators.
4. Conduct the study scrupulously and avoid confounding variables.
5. Report accurately and as soon as possible to the scientific community through a number of organs such as scholarly journals and more general publications. Get the word out to the professional and lay communities. Report your data in paper and poster presentations to as large and varied an audience as possible.

Funding is difficult at first until one has established a clearly scientific base for research and produced some results. Our suggestion is to try first for modest funding simply because it is easier to obtain. We have worked with grants as small as $1000 and $2000. Ask companies and private donors for funding close to the end of the year when everyone is looking for tax write-offs. Practice your oral presentation to a potential donor. Be certain that you are presenting the plan carefully, clearly, and without hyperbole. Justify the expenses you anticipate and show that you have looked for ways to keep the spending modest.

Our experience with federal funding is that it is cumbersome and the wait is lengthy—even if only to receive the news that you are in or out of the picture for a grant. Private donors, particularly local and regional people and foundations, are much more accessible. Federal grants tend to be run by bureaucratic minds and we wonder at times just how carefully a proposal is read. For example, a request to a federal organization for funding for the study about women in childbirth came back with a printed form indicating rejection. One of the line items for rejection was that "there was an inadequate gender representation".

We have found that presenting a specific research project that has a clear human basis and payoff to a funding source interested in that particular population or area is probably the best way of gaining attention to a project. Our current attempts are to establish a center for biofeedback and neurofeedback research and clinical study that will address the needs of the children and adults in our community who would benefit most from these services and training.

Selecting the proper journals, both scholarly and general, is crucial. Search out the most important journals in the field you are researching and write for journal guidelines for submission of manuscripts. Consider music therapy journals as well as more medically-oriented publications such as the *International Journal of Arts Medicine (IJAM)* and the *Journal of Arts In Psychotherapy*. Refer to Chapter 7 for more information about these sources.

It is also important to get your research results to the lay public. We are presently looking for popular magazines and journals that will inform the public at large about the healthful effects of lullabies on infants, the importance of relaxation and music listening and biofeedback training for pregnant women, and the comfort and distraction as well as maintained immunocompetence that music listening can give women during a dental procedure. This last is especially important for pregnant women who often avoid dental work during this period in their lives because nitrous oxide (which they often perceive as the only relief during the procedure) is contraindicated for the pregnant woman. Our message is that music listening can be as helpful as nitrous oxide during the procedure and music listening is perfectly safe.

Other important research tools are the video recorder and audiotape. These are important witnesses of the treatments and interventions used in the study. One must be scrupulous about maintaining confidentiality and obtaining permission from people who appear in these recordings. If properly done, videotapes are especially compelling evidence of changed behavior or selected physiological measure.

Our final advice is not to be afraid of research. If one begins with a simple enough project, learning takes place quickly as to what works and what does not work. One also learns the limits of resources. Research should be conducted by all professionals engaged in any aspect of music and healing. To avoid sharing gains made by using a certain protocol or procedure deprives the field of needed information. It is the professional responsibility of clinicians and researchers to make that information available.

CHAPTER 7

Basic Resources, Promotion, and Assessment

Resources

For the past four years, the Biofeedback and Neurofeedback Research Laboratory in the School of Music at Brigham Young University has conducted many studies that involve music listening. We have followed one basic concept known as the iso principle in which the music used at the onset of a session is matched to the mood of the subject. Music listening can be placed in two general categories: music that stimulates and music that is sedative. During the process of collecting and evaluating the sound materials we use in our studies, we have made the following observations:

1. The music that is most effective during biofeedback and neurofeedback training sessions has been carefully pretested with each subject to ensure that the it is indeed producing the desired physiological effect as measured by our EMG, EEG, peripheral skin temperature and EDG equipment. Our EMG machines show us decreases and increases in an aspect of muscle tension on a specific skin site. Our EEG machines show us the amplitude of brain frequency states that include delta, theta, alpha, and beta conditions. Our peripheral skin temperature machines indicate the rise and fall of temperature and, therefore, the state of relaxation of the subject. Our EDG equipment tells us about skin conductance and resistance levels of the subject.

2. There is a wide variety in taste among research subjects, which means that we offer every kind of music from Gregorian chant to country western.

3. Our resource library is continually upgraded and enlarged by adding different musical genres and styles to our collection. We add selections based on request and proven efficacy.

Through the years we have noticed that certain kinds of music and some specific artists and selections are continually requested by subjects. We offer these as a beginning, but, at the same time, we admonish our readers to do their homework and research tastes of the population and community from which they spring. Tastes in music are often regional in nature and understanding, and responding to needs is essential in building a library of viable sound materials.

**Selections Often Requested by Research Subjects,
BYU Research Lab: Sedative Music**

Classic Selections
    Adagio by Albinoni
    "Air" from *Orchestral Suite no. 3* by J. S. Bach

Adagio for Strings by Samuel Barber (This is the all-time favorite across all ages, genders, and social groups.)
"Adagio Sostenuto" from *Sonata quasi una Fantasia, op. 27 no. 2* ("Moonlight") by Beethoven
"Dance of the Blessed Spirits" from *Orpheus and Eurydice* by Gluck
"Morning" from *Peer Gynt* by Grieg
"Adagietto" from *Symphony no. 5* by Mahler
Canon by Pachelbel
"Adagio" from *String Quintet in C* by Schubert

Pop Music Selections

Enya albums. These are frequently requested by female subjects and were among the most popular with the women in our biofeedback and childbirth study.

Summer, by George Winston. This is solo piano music that was often requested by women and men.

The Wilderness Collection, Narada. Many subjects found this music restful and relaxing.

New Age music with repetitive patterns and patterns of natural sounds such as ocean waves were also popular. Albums such as these are readily available in media stores and outlets.

Instrumental religious music, particularly music recorded with string ensembles or orchestras.

Folk music, including older tunes such as the *Londonderry Air*.
Instrumental country music
Medleys of Broadway ballads
Patients' personal selections of favorite artists

Selections of Stimulative Music Used in BYU Research Studies with EEG Neurofeedback Training

100 Masterpieces, vol. 3: Wolfgang Amadeus Mozart. Laser Light Digital, 15678 Stereo, Delta Music Inc., Los Angeles, CA. The musical selections include:
Eine kleine Nachtmusik (1st movement)
Piano Concerto no. 21 in C (2nd movement)
The Marriage of Figaro (Overture)
Flute Concerto no. 2 in D (2nd movement)
Piano Sonata in A (Rondo alla Turca)
Don Giovanni (Overture)
Concerto for Horn no. 3 in E flat (2nd movement)
Piano Concerto no. 23 in A (1st movement)
The Marriage of Figaro (March)
Serenata Notturna

Other Music used in Studies Requiring Stimulative Music
Symphony no. 25 in G minor: Serenade by Mozart
Concerto for Piano no. 21 (Elvira Madigan) by Mozart

Concerto for Piano no. 22 by Mozart
Concerto for Two Pianos by Mozart
Divertimenti, (any of these are appropriate) by Mozart
Dances, Landler (any of these are appropriate) by Mozart
Symphonies (be sensitive to preferences of subjects) by Mozart
Concerti (be sensitive to preferences of subjects) by Mozart

New Age music that is highly patterned in rhythm and texture
Compositions of Handel, Haydn, Gluck, and Albinoni (again, be sensitive to preferences of subjects)

Mozart was chosen for our EEG neurofeedback studies because of the patterned rhythm in the music. The basic underlying pattern can be heard in sets of eight. The regular rhythmic patterns provide a steady beat to which subjects often directly respond. Children with Attention Deficit Disorder (ADD) often reduced their theta frequency state (displayed as vertical moving bars) in exact rhythm to the underlying beat of the background music.

Since the initial study we have used music from composers of the Classic and Baroque periods. The key is the patterned rhythm that one readily finds in this music. The order and rhythm pattern appear to enhance ability to focus and thereby improve that aspect of the subject's performance on the outcome measure.

General Guidelines for Music Listening Selections that are Sedative in Nature

Offer:
    instrumental music
    music that has a slow harmonic rhythm (changes chords slowly)
    music that has moderate dynamics and a regular repetitive rhythm
    music that relates to the age group of the subject
    music recorded with string instruments, piano, flute, harp, guitar

Check:
    effects of music on selected physiological parameters being measured, such as peripheral skin temperature increase. You can buy a monitor for a modest investment at a local electronics store.

General Guidelines for Music Listening Selections that are Stimulative in Nature

Offer:
    patterned instrumental music—music that is heard easily in sets of 8 or 10 beats
    music with a lively but moderate tempo
    music that has perceivable rhythm units the ear hears easily
    music that has moderate dynamics

music that relates to the age group of the subject
music recorded with orchestra and all types of instrumental configurations

Check:
effects of music on selected physiological parameters being measured, such as a peripheral skin temperature increase.

Other Resources
Societies
International Society for Music in Medicine (ISMM), Dr. med. Ralph Spintge, Executive Director of ISMM, Paulmannshöher Strasse 17, D-58515 Lüdenscheid, Germany.

International Arts Medicine Association (IAMA), 714 Old Lancaster Road, Bryn Mawr, PA 19010.

Society for the Arts in Healthcare (SAH), 45 Lyme Road, Suite 304, Hanover, NH 03755.

Journals
International Journal of Arts Medicine (IJAM), MMB Music, Inc., Contemporary Arts Building, 3526 Washington Avenue, Saint Louis, MO 63103-1019.

Medical Problems of Performing Artists, Hanley & Belfus, P. O. Box 1377, Philadelphia, PA 19105-9990.

Journal of Music Therapy, National Association for Music Therapy, Inc., 8455 Colesville Road, Suite 1000, Silver Spring, MD 20910.

Music Therapy, American Association for Music Therapy, 8455 Colesville Road, Suite 1000, Silver Spring, MD 20910.

Common Boundary, Common Boundary, Inc., 5272 River Road, Suite 650, Bethesda, MD 20816.

Books
The following titles are available from MMB Music, Inc., 3526 Washington Avenue, Saint Louis, MO 63103-1019 USA:

The Arts in Health Care. Edited by Charles Kaye and Tony Blee. London: Jessica Kingsley Publishers Ltd.

Book of Sound Therapy. Olivea Dewhurst-Maddock. New York, NY: Simon & Schuster, Inc.

Dance and Other Expressive Art Therapies. Edited by Fran Levy, Judith Fried, and Fern Leventhal. New York & London: Routledge.

The Handbook of Dramatherapy. Edited by Sue Jennings. New York & London: Routledge.

Healing Imagery and Music. Carol Bush. Portland, OR: Rudra Press.

Healing with Music and Color. Mary Bassano. York Beach, ME: Samuel Weiser, Inc.

Mind, Music, and Imagery. Stephanie Merritt. Santa Rosa, CA: Aslan.

Music Movement Mind and Body. Bridget Watson. Forest Knolls, CA: Elder Books.

Music Therapy with Hospitalized Children. Edited by Mary-Ann Froehlich. Cherry Hill, NJ: Jeffrey Books.

Music Therapy Research and Practice in Medicine. David Aldridge. London: Jessica Kingsley Publishers Ltd.

Musical Bridges. Joan Shaw and Carna Manthey. Saint Louis, MO: MMB Music, Inc.

MusicMedicine, volume 1. Edited by Spintge and Droh. Saint Louis, MO: MMB Music, Inc.

MusicMedicine, volume 2. Edited by Pratt and Spintge. Saint Louis, MO: MMB Music, Inc.

Play Therapy. Ann Cattanach. London: Jessica Kingsley Publishers Ltd.

Rhythmic Medicine. Janalea Hoffman. Leawood, KS: Jamillan Press.

Therapeutic Uses of Music with Older Adults. Alicia Ann Clair. Baltimore, MD: Health Professions Press, Inc.

Using the Creative Arts in Therapy. Edited by Bernie Warren. New York & London: Routledge.

Promotion

Your Hospital Arts program depends on community involvement and support. As pointed out earlier, donations of instruments and music can provide resources otherwise unavailable. Community involvement, however, goes far beyond donations; your Hospital Arts program will thrive if you have recruited volunteers from church groups, amateur and professional performing arts ensembles, and semiretired performers. The more widespread the community inclusion, the more free promotion and publicity for the program. Enthusiastic volunteers spread the word about the program and ensure an endless supply of present and future performers. This in turn saves the directors precious time and resources that can be put to better use.

Promotion Strategies

Bear in mind that this is a basic grass roots program that does not entail large and expensive promotional campaigns. Begin with free publicity. As soon as you are organized and have a track record, contact the media. This includes local papers, radio stations, and, if you are ready, television networks. We had our first television coverage by a commercial news program. After first securing permission from the hospital administration, we invited the crew to visit the stroke rehabilitation unit where we had set up a piano and convened five or six performers. We made sure that there was plenty of variety in the program and that the pieces were short and peppy. We also had some audience participation that included songs familiar to the mostly middle-aged and elderly patients. Above all, we kept the presentation on a friendly and informal basis. The reporter filmed several brief commentaries from patients and volunteers alike and the simple warmth of the program came across in the last 5 minutes finally edited down for the broadcast that evening.

Local papers love feature stories about a program such as this. There are several angles to take, including the view of the performers and the response of patients. The linking of town and gown is also of interest if the program is a direct effort of a college or university fine arts department. The best stories are those that do not dwell on or feature one or two people but catch the ambiance and spirit of the concerted effort.

Recruiting volunteers can be done by posting flyers in appropriate places on campus or in stores. Recruitment can also be done by word of mouth, asking committed volunteers to bring along another performer or to ask other interested people to contact the directors. Keep the momentum going in order to sustain the life of the program. It is a completely dynamic effort that must always be in motion in order to continue.

Design your own brochure. We chose an attractive foldout format in which we answered basic what, where, who and why questions and listed the directors' names, addresses and phone numbers. Our brochure has our own program logo and also shows the Very Special Arts logo in order to indicate our proud affiliation with our cosponsoring organization. We are presently networking with another group in a nearby city to coordinate interurban efforts and bring statewide awareness to the idea. We are also branching out into other creative arts as we discover interested artists from design, theater, and art.

Remember that the Hospital Arts idea is not proprietary. Reach out to other cities and towns and help them organize their own programs. In so doing, the idea becomes familiar to other hospitals. Always approach a friendly administrator and then get the nurses on your side; they are always the staunchest allies since they deal every day with ongoing patient care and morale. Try to help your colleagues in other groups to find funding sources and show them how to keep their expenses at a minimum.

Above all, spread out the credit. Your program will work if everyone involved feels that his or her contribution is truly valued. When and where local, regional, state, and national awards are available, you as the director must seek to nominate your volunteers individually and in groups. Keep working at the concept of a group effort. When the media cover an event or an interview, be sure to include all your directors and leaders wherever possible.

Sometimes, a local health group can be of service in putting out a snappy and attractive brochure. Approach your local health management group and ask them for ideas. Be prepared to offer evidence of the cost effectiveness of Hospital Arts. In other words, get their attention first.

You will find all of these enterprises far less daunting if you call on the talents and abilities of your directors and leaders, many of whom are very helpful in designing and promoting. Some of them may be part of families with people in advertising and promotion. By utilizing to the fullest the talents and resources of your volunteers, you remove from yourself—the chief administrator—the onus of making every choice and coming up with every idea.

CHAPTER 8

Four Models of Hospital Arts Programs

In this chapter, I will describe four models of Hospital Arts Program, all very different, and all serving important needs of patients in different stages of various illnesses. These four programs are outstanding among many examples of the creative arts in international healthcare environments. They were chosen specifically because each is unique in its thrust and is an excellent working model of healthcare givers, and a particular community. The differences in program goals, design, and implementation offer the readers variety from which to choose the best plan for their own community and situation.

Arts Medicine in an Academic Setting

Shands Hospital, a part of the University of Florida in Gainesville, created an Artists-in-Residence program in 1991. In the words of founders, John Graham-Pole, Mary Rockwood Lane, Mary Lisa Kitakis, and Leeann Stacpoole (1994), "We saw it as our overall mission to identify and develop the many connections between the creative and the healing arts in this academic medical setting" (p. 17).[1] Since there are no paid staff members, artists are drawn from the campus and community into the hospital environment.

The stated purpose of the program is to humanize the hospital environment by bringing music, dance, painting, theater, writing, puppetry, clowning, and magic into the facility and to allow caregivers opportunities to apply their own creative powers in the process. All segments of the community at large and in the institution are included in the program. The idea is to utilize the creative arts to bring patients, artists, and caregivers together.

The Artists-in-Residence program was begun in the Bone Marrow Transplant Unit, an 18-bed facility that accommodates six children and six to twelve adults. Ninety percent of the patients have advanced cancer. This unit was chosen because these patients and families have the greatest need. Treatments are invasive, extended, and painful, and periods of hospitalization often seem interminable.

The Artists-in-Residence program quickly spread to other units and the program directors report that there are currently 14 visual, literary, and performance artists in the facility working 4–20 hours per week. They have found that it works best to build a critical mass in each unit instead of relying on one artist.

When one enters the atrium of Shands Hospital, the most striking distinction between this area and that of other institutions is the presence of several

---

[1]Graham-Pole et al. (1994, Winter). Creating an arts program in an academic medical setting. *IJAM*, 3(2), 17–25.

Healing Walls, comprised of ceramic tiles on which patients have painted their personal expressions of feelings associated with their illness. The effect is stunning and also very moving as one reads the messages, both pictorial and written on the tiles. The latest venture is to paint 12-inch square ceiling panels. So far over 1000 have been painted by patients, families, and staff and placed in the hospital's ceiling.

John Graham-Pole, the physician among the directors, is a pediatric oncologist who is also a clown, dresses up in the most outlandish costumes, and has a most unusual business card. To the children, these moments of lightness and silliness are vital in maintaining a perspective on life and healing. There is still something to smile about, especially if it involves aiming a missile at your doctor during a marshmallow fight—a phenomenon not unknown on the unit. Other physicians have created an ensemble known as the Docs of Dixie, a group that performs Dixieland jazz for resident audiences in the hospital. Dancers take patients as partners and artists create canvases, tiles, collages, and the like with children and adults. Musicians play for individual patients or for groups of listeners. A Rabbi's wife visits frequently to tell stories to children. In other words, a concerted effort has been made to reach every resource in the human community to share talent with children and adults.

The key factor in the success of this program is a physician who not only allows the creative arts in the units he oversees, but actually encourages their inclusion in daily activities. Dr. Graham-Pole is such a human being who has never permitted the seriousness of his duties and responsibility to compromise

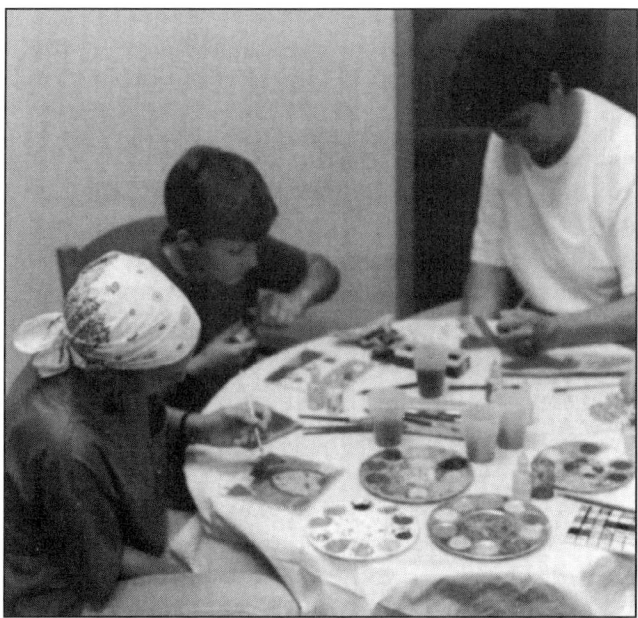

Patients, families, and artists working together

his inherent sense of humor and sensitive spirit. He codirects Arts in Medicine (AIM) with a nurse-painter, Mary Rockwood Lane, who will shortly complete her Ph.D. dissertation based on this program. The first AIM conference, held in June 1995 at Shands Hospital, demonstrated to all participants the power of the arts in a hospital setting.

Dr. Graham-Pole says that he wanted to create AIM in order to bring more creativity into his own life. The release of human creative expression among children and adults in various stages of pain and physical ravage is a unique tool to be used alongside the medicines and treatments that accompany serious illness. Although Dr. Graham-Pole is the reason this particular program has developed, it would not have come into being without the talents and willingness of the nurses and artists who assisted him in this work. The overall success factor then is team spirit and work and generous use of talent available at the professional and community levels.

Contact person for the Shands Hospital Artists-in-Residence program:

>John Graham-Pole, M.D.
>Dept. of Pediatrics
>University of Florida
>Gainesville, FL 32610
>Phone: (352) 395-0114
>Fax: (352) 338-9808
>email: jgp.peds@mail.health.ufl.edu

Music Medicine in a Clinic for Patients with Cancer

The Medical Clinic III is part of the Ludwig-Maximilians-Universität, Klinikum Grosshadern, Munich, Germany. Under the supervision of the clinic's Director, Prof. Dr. W. Wilmanns, a pilot project is underway that uses music as a palliative adjunct during chemotherapy. The psychologist-music therapist involved in this project is Ms. Susan Weber.

Cancer patients are confronted with a double trauma, namely, the diagnosis of cancer and the prospect of ongoing therapy. Even if they view the therapy positively as lifesaving, at the onset they often experience high anxiety and uncertainty concerning side effects and outcome. When a patient is in remission, there is always the fear that the disease may return; when this happens, patients are even more overwrought because they know what awaits them. The introduction of music listening at this point has been helpful in mitigating some of this anxiety.

According to psychologist-music therapist Susan Weber, the music program (under the joint direction of a psychologist-music therapist, and an oncologist) has been easily worked into the routine of the oncology ward. Patients interested in the program are given a questionnaire that focuses on their physical and emotional well-being and musical preferences.

During an interview with the psychologist-music therapist, patients set personal goals that include anxiety reduction, relaxation, and mood improvement. Patients may select CDs from a wide variety of musical genres and styles and then listen to the music as they use strategies that include visualization and other activities. The categories from which they can choose include classical, light orchestral, German Volksmusik, pop, light rock, big band, and the like. The clinic has approximately 400 CDs. The patient is then given his own portable player, his selected CDs, and instructed in the proper use of the equipment. The protocol is to ask the patient to begin listening to his selected music 15 minutes before chemotherapy treatment is started. From there, patients decide how long they will continue to listen to the music during their treatment, which may last from several hours to weeks, including a period in isolation. Following the chemotherapy, patients are asked to (a) evaluate the use of music by responding to a questionnaire and (b) state their wishes for future treatments. Music is an on-the-spot adjunctive tool for which patients need no previous counseling or training to participate.

Within the last 2 years, 75 patients have chosen to listen to music. Those who did wanted to continue using the music and reported that it provided diversion, relaxation, and the opportunity to forget the therapy, at least temporarily. These patients also reported less tension, improved quality in the hospital stay, better coping skills, and a sense of well-being. Ninety percent of the patients requested classical music during the actual chemotherapy treatment, although they listened to other types in between if the stay was prolonged. Piano and guitar were preferred over other solo instruments or larger symphonic settings. Mozart was the most requested composer, followed by choices of classical CDs specifically produced for relaxation purposes. Music helps in other ways, such as a distractor when chemotherapy was delayed, or an aid while being hooked up to the equipment, or a way to block out unwanted thoughts or

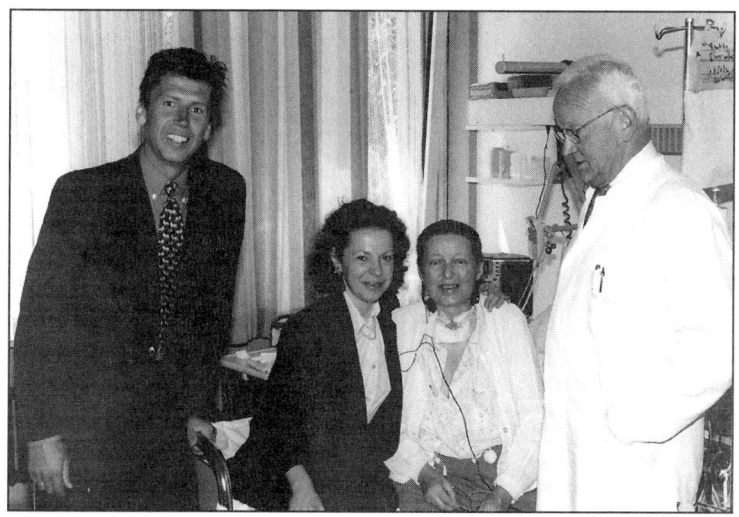

Dr. Volkmar Nüssler, Susan Weber, Mrs. Gisela Barth, and Dr. Wolfgang Wilmanns

events. It also helps patients get through the night, cope with an agitated roommate, alleviate loneliness, bounce back, reestablish more hopeful outlooks, and get in contact with inner spiritual resources.

Patients who return for more chemotherapy treatments still have anxiety but are relieved to know that music is still there for their use. The project is being continued and will be subjected to a more scientific evaluation by adding a control group and testing patients' parameters of immunity. Resources for the program include a wide selection of CDs and portable players. The variety of musical offerings is necessary because it is advisable to avoid using the same music for subsequent treatments in order to prevent patient association of one particular music with chemotherapy treatment. The services of a psychologist-music therapist are important because, in addition to needing someone familiar with the psychological components of patient anxiety and stress, knowledge of musical repertoire is also vital.

Contact persons for the program are:

>Dr. Volkmar Nüssler
>Bruckenfischerstrasse 7
>81547 Munich, Germany
>Phone: 089 6900194
>Fax: 089 7004418
>email: nuessler@gsf.de
>
>Susan Weber, M.A.
>Clemenstrasse 84
>80796 Munich, Germany
>Phone: 089 303137
>Fax: 089 301259
>email: swebermuc@aol.com

Hospital Arts—A University-Community Project

The Hospital Arts Program, cosponsored by Arts Access/Utah, Very Special Arts; and the School of Music, Brigham Young University, was created in 1993 in Provo, Utah. The original idea, conceived by Rosalie Rebollo Pratt, Professor of Music, Brigham Young University, was to organize student volunteers to visit the stroke unit at Utah Valley Regional Medical Center. The first student Codirectors of the program included Kristin Weber, Jacquelyn M. Coleman, and Camille Hillam.

Consisting of some six performing majors and their faculty advisor, the first volunteers visited the administrators of the facility and asked if they could bring some live music into the hospital. The administrative staff of the hospital were extremely receptive and a plan was worked out that would meet the needs of both the hospital residents and the students. Students were interviewed and given photo IDs. Next, they were briefed about hospital routines, the best times and places for visits, and the kinds of music and instruments that would best suit the patients and the environment.

The very first visit was made on a Sunday evening at 5:30 by the entire group of volunteers to patients who had congregated in the common dining area of the stroke unit. An upright piano had been wheeled into the area and the first selection was a hymn suggested by one of the patients. Since Provo is a largely Mormon community, the choice was logical and gave all present an opportunity to participate. By the time the evening ended at 6:30, the six students had moved among all the patients, most of whom were wheelchair bound. Names were learned and small talk was exchanged about backgrounds and interests. Patients also expressed their preferences for music to be played and sung at the next visit. Since the patient population was largely 55 years old and above, many of the song titles were golden oldies.

Students learned to use fake books, sing with patients, and accept responses at all levels. The nurses on the unit were particularly interested in encouraging patients to sing because it helped those who needed speech practice. Our singers and instrumentalists also learned to work with an audience of people who have suffered varying degrees of physical and emotional damage. Many patients did not respond in ways that were familiar to the musicians, such as clapping or showing verbal enthusiasm for the performances. Some patients even wept openly and profusely as the music was played. Nurses explained that emotions of these patients are often close to the surface and tears are easily generated. Our youngest patient in the unit was a 14-year-old girl who had suffered a stroke two years prior to her admission to this hospital. After a month of visits, the girl got up one evening and began to dance—something she had not done since her stroke.

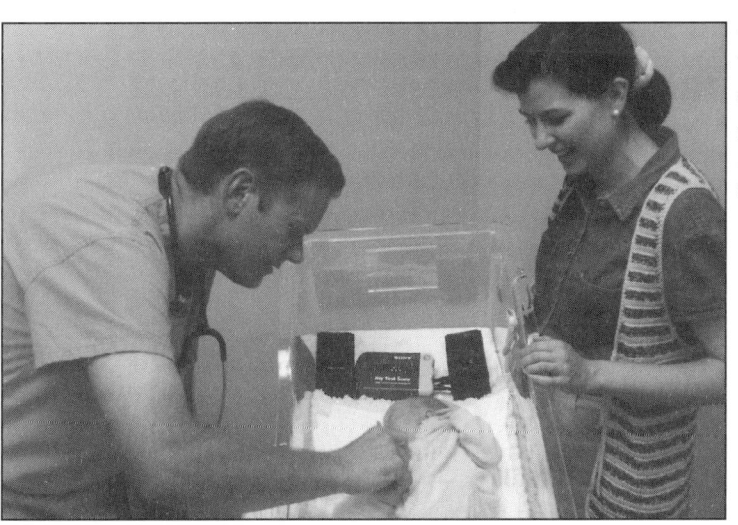

Dr. Ronald Stoddard, an infant in the Premature Intensive Care Unit, and Jacquelyn M. Coleman

The student volunteer ranks grew quickly as word got around the BYU School of Music. Students were able to sign up for 1 hour of credit, for which they visited the hospital once a week and kept a journal of their experiences with patients and staff. By the end of the year, the program was listed with United Way and community members joined the group. We also expanded the program to include one-on-one visits to patients who were unable to leave their rooms. These patients, most of whom were on the telemetry unit, were visited by a musician who asked if they were interested in hearing some music or singing a favorite song. Almost everyone who was asked was eager to welcome the musician and listen to at least 10 minutes of music. Patients in a weakened condition could tolerate about this much time before they needed to rest. Students soon became sensitive to this need and were quick to shorten a visit when the patient was tired. Many patients, however, appeared to be invigorated by the music and were especially happy to join in a song whenever possible.

In 1994, we had the great luck of being noticed by Art Access/Very Special Arts Utah, the Utah affiliate of the international organization Very Special Arts, a program of the Kennedy Center, Washington, DC. Ruth Lubbers, the Executive Director of the program visited Provo that year and observed the work we were doing in the hospital and the program we had begun at some local retirement homes. She then designated us as a special district program and we began to receive funding each year. With this generous support we developed brochures, retained several student administrators, and expanded the program to include the State hospital. Our program in the local Seville Retirement Home is very popular with the residents and we perform every Sunday afternoon with music of every genre and style. We have visited a high school for unwed mothers, a shelter for children in crisis, and have made a short video of the program. We will also be able with these funds to bring international creative arts experts to visit our program.

Our keys to success are our wonderful student Codirectors, Kristin Weber, Jacqueline M. Coleman, and Camille Hillam, whose energy and enthusiasm have built and sustained the entire program. Our student musicians, the backbone of the performance component of the program, develop new understanding of the value of their art and its impact on populations within the society that are usually not considered part of the traditional concert audience.

Contact person for the program is:

> Dr. Rosalie Rebollo Pratt
> C550 Harris Fine Arts Center
> Brigham Young University
> Provo, Utah 84603
> Phone: (801) 378-6341
> Fax: (801) 226-6642
> email: rrpratt@byu.edu

Cultural Services Program at Duke University Medical Center

Janice B. Palmer is the director of the Cultural Services Program at the Duke University Medical Center in Durham, North Carolina. One of the oldest examples in arts in healthcare, the Cultural Services program received funding in 1978 from the Mary Duke Biddle Foundation and the National Endowment for the Arts to begin a collaboration with the Durham Arts Council to explore the role of the arts and humanities in modern healthcare. Ms. Palmer is also one of the founders of the Society for the Arts in Healthcare (SAH), which maintains an arts in healthcare database and hosts annual conferences. Both Janice Palmer and Florence Nash have written the *Hospital Arts Handbook* that is a wealth of information for those who are interested in beginning a similar program in their communities.

Cultural Services' mission is to integrate the arts and humanities into the life of the Medical Center, bringing the healing power of the arts to people who are suffering and to those who care for them, including staff and students. Cultural Services' first project was the acquisition of original art by North Carolina artists for patient rooms. There are now more than 1,200 originals throughout the hospital, including 92 quiltings by 24 North Carolina quiltmakers on the ob-gyn unit. The placement of art in public areas led to a close collaboration with the Medical Center's facilities design office to bring the artist's perspective into public spaces such as entries, lobbies, and courtyards. Most recently, this perspective has extended to the design of landscaping and special gardens for the Medical Center campus. Past projects include birdhouses made by Appalachian craftsmen in the pediatric playyard, newspaper vending machines in a courtyard selling newspaper-sized, artist-designed get well cards, and 500 life-sized clay tiles of birds on the walls of a two-story courtyard that also held eight 10-foot tall "bird lanterns". Present planning includes a fragrance garden for the Eye Center with the paving and seating designed by two artists. All of these projects help increase the patient's sense of control, access to social support, and positive distractions in the physical environment. Familiarity and comfort replace alienation and fear. Involvement of the creative arts in redesigning the hospital facility and grounds includes items such as signage, lighting, wall covering, and painting, as well as sculpture and the presence of dancers, musicians, storytellers, and poets strolling through wards and patients' rooms. This arrangement offers artists access to a population for which they had not previously performed or created.

The Cultural Services program includes a group known as the Osler Literary Roundtable, named after Sir William Osler, who, like Heraclitus and Galen, advocated the cultivation of the arts and humanities in physician training and practice. The group began as an opportunity for employees, doctors, students, and friends from all over the hospital to meet weekly and read and discuss contemporary literature. Short stories, novels, poems and the like are talked about as participants eat their lunches. The Roundtable has sponsored three poetry contests, open to anyone having any connection with the Medical Center. Pro-

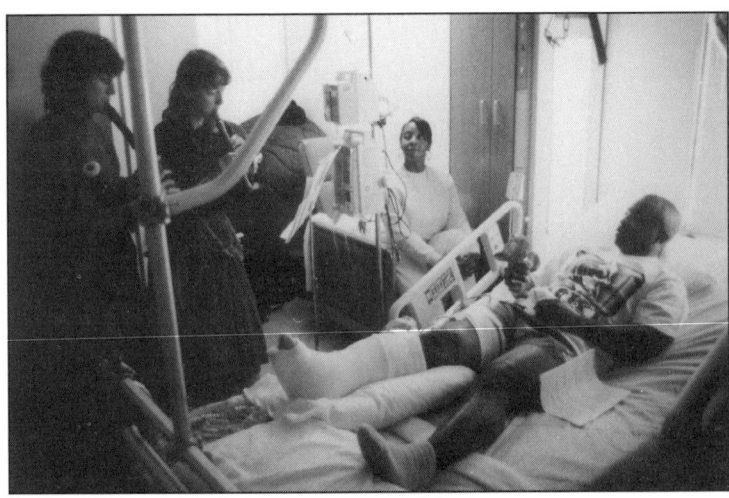

A room service performance. Musicians go from door to door offering patients and their families a little musical interlude.

fessional poets have judged each contest, and awards are given. In addition, all the poems (more than 100 in the last contest) are displayed in the hospital and then printed in a small paperback book. The most remarkable outcome of the contest was the revelation that healthcare providers and receivers had deeply felt emotions that poured forth from people as different as so-called emotionless physicians, grieving relatives, nurses and aides who needed this conduit for expression of feelings they had never voiced in poetry.

The Center now has a closed-circuit television system that includes an Arts and Humanities Channel on which films and videotapes by and about North Carolina artists are broadcast. An electronic bulletin board alerts patients to a variety of artistic offerings in the community.

In addition to bringing the arts into medicine, medicine is also brought into the arts, which can include the examination of performance-related injuries. In 1989, the Nancy Hanks Artist-in-Residence was the dancer Jacques D'Amboise, who talked with medical students about what dancers need from the healthcare system. All of this effort helps to rehumanize the healthcare environment in the spirit of early physicians such as Hippocrates and Galen, both of whom believed in holistic care of patients who were to be diagnosed and treated as whole persons. Ms. Palmer is pleased with the fact that there are physicians at the Center who are taking seriously the notion of the creative arts in a healthcare environment. In her own words: "People from all phases of life come to the hospital. And we are the largest employer in the county, with 8000 people. When you look at it that way, you could say we're running an arts council for a small community."

Contact person for the program is:

> Ms. Janice Palmer
> DUMC, 3017
> Durham, North Carolina 27710
> Phone: (919) 286-3361
> Fax: (919) 286-7907
> email: palme008@mc.duke.edu